The Smile Owner's Manual

Let me start off by saying, my dental anxiety is pretty bad. So bad that I've avoided the dentist for a little over ten years... My first visit I walked in crying due to being in a lot of pain, everyone was super nice and caring and eased my worries. Dr. Sykes was very kind and talked me through everything including different treatment plans/costs. After that Emergency visit I felt very comfortable and taken care of by everyone at The Reno Dentist so much that I decided to make them my home base for dentistry and started with a dental plan to get on track with my oral health. I've gone back to the Reno Dentist since my first Emergency visit and as soon as I walked in they remembered my name, little things about my life that we talked about and it was the same happy, genuine welcome from everyone who worked there. I highly recommend The Reno Dentist for all your dental care! They are Great!

Google Review from C. J.

Dr Sykes and his staff are the friendliest and best dentist place I have ever been to in my 50 years of getting dental work. They really care and are sincerely concerned about you and whatever problem you might be going through at the time. If you ever change your dentist, you won't be sorry for going to see Dr Sykes. Thank you for taking care of me.

Google Review from M.

First time in the office and had a great experience. All the needed treatments were explained very well. Was also given all the information needed to continue all my dental needs.

Google Review from G. B.

What Patients Are Saying

They are best dentist I have ever had, definitely life changing. they took me as emergency and couldn't have asked for a better experience, I am now in the process of a smile makeover and they are always willing to make things work best for me and my life. Is it weird to have a new found love for going to the dentist? I am not scared anymore! Highly recommend for anyone who is struggling with getting themselves to go to the dentist, you will be comfortable here!

Google Review from S. T.

I am blown away each appointment I have. EVERYONE is so friendly and helpful. Everything has been so wonderful. What a great environment!

Google Review from K. A.

First time I can say I went to a dentist and had a good experience. Amazing staff.

Google Review from K.

Love this place. Everyone from the front desk to the hygienist to the doctors are incredibly kind and professional. I don't mind the long drive from home at all- the experience is worth the time. Thank you guys!

Google Review from J. A.

I have never had a more caring, compassionate dentist in my life. Dr Sykes is an amazing dentist that I would recommend over and over. Not only has he and his whole office make me feel comfortable (I hated dentists before this), but he remembers each of his patients and truly CARES about them. I am beyond grateful for finding this office.

Google Review from C. R.

Bad timing on my part, not having the dental insurance. HOWEVER, I absolutely could not wait another hour and this office was top notch, they were able to remove my cursed, rotting tooth the same day and the Dentist and staff were absolutely wonderful. Everyone including myself left their office smiling which was a good sign, and Dr. Adams was very personable and kind which I appreciated. Took less than 10mins to remove it once the meds kicked in. Left their office pain free and healing went great! I didn't even need extra pain meds. 2 weeks later and it's fully healed up and naturally sealed up. Thank you!

Google Review from C. C.

The Reno Dentist are awesome!! I'm a long haul truck driver and needed dental help. They got me in right away and got me out of pain. Every single person in the office is very nice and professional. It was refreshing to get such good, prompt and professional service. If you need a dentist in Reno give them a call.

Google Review from M. O.

My husband is very dentist-averse, and this is the first office he has willingly visited. Dr. Sykes and Dr. Adams have done amazing work, removing broken teeth and rebuilding his smile. Thank you so much, we love you all!!!

Google Review from R. P.

A truly amazing experience. They are state of the art. I needed a rather tricky Crown. They used a Laser to trim my gums and I was able to watch a computer guided machine craft my Crown and cook it in just 45 minutes. I was in and out with a new Crown in 90 minutes.

Google Review from D. T.

I went here for a problem I was having with a root canal. I came here for the first time and the doctor was absolutely amazing!!!!! He knew exactly what he was doing! I will be coming here for my cleanings and any problems I have with my teeth for the time left I have in Nevada!!! Love it here, I highly recommend this doctor as I am a super picky person.

Google Review from L. P.

They were great! Super fast, painless, and helpful! From the moment I walked in to the minute I left they made me feel like I mattered!

Google Review from B. D.

An amazing staff the created a welcoming, comfortable environment. The procedure was straightforward and I was given all the necessary and available information. It was a quick and pleasant visit and the Doctors really make it an effort to take care of you as a patient.

Google Review from A. M.

I haven't been to dentist for more then 20 years so I was a little nervous. I was so happy with my appointment and excited to finally get a beautiful white smile again . Dr Sykes even called and checked on me the next day I was so happy! Thank Dr. Sykes and everyone to the hygienist to assistants and all staff . I'm so excited to be getting a beautiful smile .

Google Review from L. B.

The Smile Owner's Manual

A SIMPLE GUIDE TO UNDERSTANDING AND IMPROVING YOUR SMILE

Shane Sykes, DMD

DISCLAIMER

Regardless of how close to your face you are holding this book, I can't see your teeth and I cannot give you advice tailored to your specific needs--but I can share two decades of experience in helping my patients smile confidently

CONTENTS

Bonus Content

INTRODUCTION

Dear Reader,

This book is written as an informational tool to help you make educated and informed decisions improving your smile. The chapters of this book are designed to give you the information you need to understand the options available in dentistry today and the real-world pros and cons of each of those options. We start with the assumption that you have a basically healthy mouth and that you're considering cosmetic enhancement. Health comes first and cosmetics build upon that. I suggest that you read Part One of the book first and then browse through the book learning about solutions to your specific concerns. The chapters are arranged from less invasive to more invasive dental treatments. I prefer conservative treatments, but sometimes invasive treatment is a more appropriate option. Scattered throughout the book are stories from my clinical experience. All these stories are true (but the names and identifying details have been changed to protect individuals' privacy).

Use the following table to focus your reading on the treatments that are most likely to resolve your concerns.

At the end of the book there is bonus content about:

- How to choose a dentist,
- How to maximize your dental insurance,
- Seeking dental care abroad.

Dental Concern	Chapters to Read
Crooked teeth	8, 11, 12, 13, 15, 19
Gaps between teeth	8, 11, 13, 15
Broken teeth	8, 12, 13, 15, 19, 20
Yellow or discolored teeth	9, 13, 14, 15
Missing teeth	8, 17, 18, 19, 20
"Buck teeth"	11, 12, 15, 19, 20
Misshapen teeth	10, 12, 13, 15, 19
Ugly teeth	1-21
Puffy gums or bad breath	10
Gummy smile	10
My teeth don't show when I smile	8, 11, 13, 15, 19
I want some bling!	21
Old, ugly fillings	9, 13, 14, 15
Black teeth	9, 14, 15
Worn or chipped teeth	19

Part 1

Science

Shane Sykes, DMD

1 -- WHY DO WE SMILE?

One day during my bicycle commute to work I felt particularly happy--so I smiled at all the oncoming cars, joggers, and people out working in their yards. Surprisingly, most of them looked around sheepishly, then smiled and waved at me. Without any verbal communication we had made an emotional connection in just milli-seconds of interaction. We silently said to each other "I see you and recognize your value. Thanks for being you!"

As the days went by and I continued my smiley commute, I began to develop friendships with strangers I've never met--the security guard outside the bank; the older cyclist on 4th street that I can never keep up with; the woman with the cute white dog and the immaculate rose garden. We made a bond and looked forward to seeing each other. We created a connection--simply by smiling.

I'm not the first to recognize the power of our smiles. In addition to his famous Theory of Evolution, Charles Darwin developed a complex theory about how smiling and laughing influences the physiology of our minds and bodies. He advanced the *Facial Feedback Response Theory*, which suggests that the act of smiling can make us feel better when we're down, instead of being something that we do when we *already* feel good.

Centuries later, an intriguing 30-yearlong study at UC Berkeley[1] examined the smiles of students in an old yearbook and measured their well-being and success throughout their lives. By measuring the relative size of smiles in the photographs the researchers successfully predicted--how fulfilling and long lasting their marriages would be; how highly they would score on standardized tests of well-being and general happiness; and how inspiring they would be to others. The widest smilers consistently ranked highest in all three areas.

In a fascinating study[2] two professors looked back at the 1952 baseball cards photos of Major League players. The professors found that the span of a player's smile could predict the span of his life! Players who didn't smile in their pictures lived an average of 72.9 years, while players with beaming smiles lived an average of 79.9 years.

Perhaps not surprisingly, we're *born* smiling. 3-D ultrasound technology shows that developing babies appear to smile even in the womb. After they're born, babies continue to smile (initially mostly in their sleep) and even blind babies[3] smile in response to the sound of the human voice.

Smiles are one of the most basic, biologically uniform expressions of all humans. Paul Ekman (the world's leading expert on facial expressions) documented[4] that smiles are cross-cultural and have the same meaning in different societies. In studies he conducted in Papua New Guinea, Ekman found that members of the Fore tribe--who were completely disconnected from outside cultures and were known for their unusual cannibalistic rituals--used smiles the same way you and I would. A smile means the same thing to all of us!

Smiling is not just a universal means of communicating, it's also a frequent one. Many of us smile more than 20 times a day and few people smile less than 5 times a day. Have you ever wondered why being around children makes you smile more often? Those with the greatest smiling superpowers are actually children--who smile and laugh[5] as many as 300 times per day!

Several studies in Sweden[6] confirmed that other people's smiles suppress the control we usually have over our own facial muscles, compelling us to smile. Our Swedish friends also showed that it's very difficult to frown when looking at someone who smiles. Why? Because smiling is evolutionarily contagious, and we have a subconscious innate drive to smile when we see someone smiling. This occurs even among strangers when we have no intention to connect or affiliate with the other person, like I experienced on my smiley bike commutes. In fact, I bet you're smiling right now just reading this--or at least you are now! Mimicking a smile and experiencing it physically helps us interpret how genuine a smile is. This helps us understand the real emotional state of the smile giver, and also positively influences our own emotional state.

In a very clever experiment[7] people were asked to evaluate real vs. fake smiles while holding a pencil in their mouths to block the muscles that help us smile. Without the pencils in their mouths, people were excellent judges of others' emotions, but with the pencils clenched between their teeth--thus preventing them from mimicking the smiles they saw--they were not very good judges of others emotions.

Smiling even has an influence on our brain chemistry. Scientists have used fMRI testing[8] to measure brain activity after injecting Botox to suppress mouth muscle and showed that facial feedback (such as imitating a smile) changes how our brain sees emotions. This demonstrates that our brain's happiness-wiring is switched on when we smile!

Additionally, smiling has many therapeutic effects[9] and has been associated with--reducing harmful stress hormones, increasing health-enhancing hormones, and lowering blood pressure.

If all these benefits are still not enough, smiling also makes us look good in the eyes of others. One Penn State University study confirmed that when we smile, we not only appear more likeable and courteous, but we're actually perceived to be more competent. My own personal experiments have also revealed that people who smile get better customer service and have shorter wait-times in line. Once I was traveling back to the USA with my wife and six children. As we stood in the seemingly endless queue of travelers snaking back and forth while waiting to clear customs, I happened to make eye contact with a customs employee. Out of conscious habit I smiled at her and she smiled back. She looked around briefly and then walked over to me. To my surprise she lifted the retractable fabric barrier off the post near us, set it aside and invited us to step out of line. After closing the barrier, she said, "Welcome home, please follow me," and escorted us directly to an available customs agent--bypassing the agonizing 45-minute wait to get through customs. All thanks to a simple smile!

So far, we have only discussed the benefits of *using* your smile. Note that none of the above research evaluated the cosmetic *quality* of smiles, just the fact of smiling vs. not smiling. Now let's look briefly at the benefits of *improving* your smile. While studying at the University of Kentucky I conducted a study in which we measured the self-esteem of patients before and after undergoing major cosmetic dental treatment, or "smile makeovers." Past research[10] has shown that the single greatest predictor of self-esteem is how we feel about our appearance, and the most significant contributor to that is how we feel about our mouth, eyes, and hair. I found a statistically significant improvement in people's overall self-esteem after improving just their smile. Changing our smiles *can* change our lives.

Unfortunately, with the ever-increasing pressure of social media we can also fall prey to great unhappiness in the pursuit of perfection. In my practice I have helped patients who were unhappy because they didn't like their smile. After extensive work to give them a gorgeous smile, sometimes I was sad to see that although they were now happy with their smile, they had become unhappy with their nose, or their eyes, or some other aspect of their appearance. There is an addiction in the pursuit of perfection that can never be satisfied. This is called Body Dysmorphic Disorder. It is important that as a society we acknowledge and discuss this problem. We must learn to recognize our own beauty and value regardless of any imperfections we may view within ourselves. I love the message of Madilyn Paige's song "Perfect"--

"Take a picture, dress it up
Keep the best and crop it out
All she wants to be
Is something to see
Hide the scars and hide the flaws
Fitting in is all she wants
She needs to be
More than she sees
Oh, the games we think we have to play
To make us feel a certain way
We'll never win with all of this
Obsession with perfect,
Lost in misdirection
Obsession with perfect,
Twisted our reflections
We're already worth it,
'Cause worth is not a prize you can win or lose
You're already worth it
Let go, let go
Let go of perfect"

It is also important to consider the difference between genuine and forced smiles. We know that when you genuinely smile you look and feel good, and our smiles are contagious and can make others feel good too. But it is important to note that this primarily applies to *genuine* smiles. While some research suggests positive emotional benefits with fake or forced smiles, a 2019 study[11] found significant negative consequences (like increased alcohol consumption) among people who fake a smile too much.

So, if you want to feel rich, live longer, reduce stress or wait less in line--begin connecting with those around you by sharing a big, genuine smile. Smile regardless of how perfect or quirky your teeth are. You'll feel better and you'll bless others. Perhaps this is why Mother Teresa said, "I will never understand all the good that a simple smile can accomplish."

2 -- THE BEAUTY OF TEETH

What do you want from your smile? What makes a smile beautiful? Your mouth has many functional and esthetic purposes. In addition to the many social purposes of smiling, you use your mouth to eat and speak. These functions have tremendously different structural needs. For proper speaking the relationship between the lips, the biting edges of the teeth, and the position of the tongue need to fit within minutely specific parameters. For ideal chewing function the upper and lower teeth should mesh together like cogs on a gear, and the teeth should be shaped with intricate peaks and valleys to manage the tremendous forces of chewing--some people can bite with up to 400 pounds of force!

The architect Louis Henry Sullivan said, "Form follows function." When the structural elements of a healthy jaw system come together in harmony, we perceive the result as a beautiful smile. Functional things are beautiful, and beautiful things are functional. Evolutionarily, we are attracted to characteristics that are strong, virile, and durable. We call these things "beautiful."

Another aspect of physical beauty is symmetry. When the left and right sides of a person's face or body are not symmetrical it suggests an underlying problem. A study[12] using computer-generated faces revealed that better left/right symmetry is more appealing and sexually attractive.

Today media, cinema, and social media play a disproportionate role in what we perceive as beautiful. We are inundated with images of what the world tells us is beautiful and what the world says we should look like. There may be some evolutionary basis to the current trends, but much of it is artificial and unnatural. Even some supermodels admit that they hardly recognize the photoshopped images of themselves.

After two decades of study, research, and clinical experience in changing people's smiles I believe that although there are many social and physical characteristics that contribute to a beautiful smile, ultimately beauty comes from confidence. If you feel good about yourself, if you feel satisfied with who you are--you are beautiful!

3 -- WHAT DO YOU WANT?

Let's talk about what you want! What do you see in your smile that you would like to change? More importantly, why do you want to change that? What do you want that change to do for you? I have had many patients say "I want veneers," but I have never had a patient say "I would like a thin layer of semi-translucent porcelain bonded over the enamel on my teeth to restore the fractured enamel and mask excessive chroma," which is what veneers do. Instead of saying what you want--"I want veneers"--you need to understand why you want it. For example, "I want to feel confident for my wedding photos and changing the shape and color of my front teeth will do that for me." There are usually several options to get to the same result, and one option will be better than another depending on your underlying motivation.

Next, consider how close your smile is relative to what you want. Does your smile need to change, or does your perception of your smile need to change for you to get you what you want? Occasionally I'll have a beautiful patient come to me complaining that they hate their smile, that their teeth are ugly because they are see-through and not white enough. Often, when I show them the color-guide we use to measure the whiteness of teeth they point to the second whitest color and say, "I don't want my teeth to look fake or too white, so I like this color." Then when we measure the current color of their teeth, they realize their teeth are already that color. They are thrilled! When I further explain that the shape of their teeth and the see-through appearance of the biting edge is natural and is exactly what we try to recreate when we make veneers the patient becomes excited. In the end I tell them, "You have a beautiful smile. If I were forced to do a smile makeover on your mouth, I would take a photo of your current smile and do everything I could to recreate it in your new smile." Sometimes just educating ourselves about what is natural and healthy is enough to give us peace of mind and confidence in our appearance. **In some cases, changing our perception is more effective than changing our teeth**.

It is important to point out that teeth are not mandatory for a happy, healthy life. Yes, teeth are helpful for ideal speech and chewing function, but there are millions of people who live wonderful lives without any teeth.

George's Story

I always felt that everyone needed teeth for eating, even if they were dentures-- then I met George. George came to me in his mid-forties asking if I would make denture for him. He said that

---

George's Story - cont.

he had all his teeth pulled when he was twenty years old and has never worn or wanted to wear dentures. But now he was a candidate for a promotion at work and he needed a better smile to help close the deal.

"Hold on and back up a moment" I interrupted him. "For twenty years you haven't had anything to chew with? How well can you eat?" I asked, perplexed.

"Perfectly fine!" he replied, smiling broadly.

"Can you eat raw vegetables?" I asked, assuming I knew more about his 20 years of toothless life than he did!

"Absolutely, love 'em." He grinned with a mischevious gleam in his eye.

"Steak?" I asked defensively.

"Tri-tip is my favorite!" he boxed back.

"Peanuts?" I countered, sure I had him cornered this time.

"Yes, but I prefer almonds." He jabbed his final blow.

I was astounded, George changed my paradigm of what is necessary for satisfaction and good nutrition. I'm sure he doesn't chew his food as finely as he could with teeth or dentures, but he is fit and trim and doesn't live on a diet of soft, processed foods. I told him that I would be happy to make him teeth to improve his smile and help secure a job promotion, but that I expected he would take the dentures out to eat.

4 – THE FIVE COSMETIC PREREQUISITES

For a smile to be beautiful and lasting it must be healthy. This book assumes that your whole "chewing system" is healthy. When evaluating a patient's dental health I prioritize the following areas of health:

1. Oral cancer
2. Gum health
3. Airway and sleep apnea
4. Clenching and grinding
5. Chewing function

It is essential to achieve health in all these areas in order to have a lasting, beautiful smile.

1 - Oral cancer is one of the most difficult and deadly cancers still today. Only about half of the people diagnosed with oral cancer survive more than five years, and it kills one person per hour, every day of the year. Fortunately, with proper and regular oral cancer screenings we can detect the precursor tissue changes or detect the cancer while it is small. **Because oral cancer can mimic something as simple as a bite**

on the inside of your cheek, it is important to have any sore or discolored area of your mouth looked at by a professional if it does not heal within 14 days.

2 - Healthy gums are important for a beautiful smile not only because the delicately contoured pink gums accentuate the beauty of your teeth, but because they provide the foundation that supports the teeth. Gingivitis is a common infection and inflammation of the visible gums. Gingivitis makes the gums red, puffy, and they bleed easily. Deeper infection of the gums is called periodontitis, or Periodontal Disease. Periodontal Disease is the number one cause of tooth loss today. It is caused by bacteria deep in the gum pockets around the roots. The bacteria destroys the bone supporting the teeth, resulting in shifting and loose teeth. Not only is it critical to make sure the foundation of your smile is healthy before doing any work to improve your smile, making your gums healthy will extend your life! Periodontal Disease is linked to preterm delivery of babies, various cancers, and **new research has shown that gum infection can actually *cause* you to have a heart attack or stroke.**

3 - Sleep apnea is a silent killer. Simply put, it is a condition where you stop breathing in your sleep for ten seconds or more--sometimes up to a full minute-- many times each hour. As you can imagine, this takes a tremendous toll on the brain, the body, and wreaks havoc on sleep quality. Most people who have sleep apnea don't even know it. They just feel tired during the day, or have headaches in the morning, and almost always have high blood pressure. If you have untreated sleep apnea it is nearly impossible to lose weight. Not everyone with sleep apnea snores, but around half of

people who snore also have sleep apnea. Oxygen deprivation, obesity, and high blood pressure put you at much higher risk of having a heart attack, a stroke, or falling asleep at the wheel and causing a deadly car crash. Sleep breathing problems cause severe sleep disruption for bed partners as well and often leads to a sleep divorce--where couples feel the only solution is to sleep in separate bedrooms. The times when I have been able to help change someone's life the most dramatically have been related to treating sleep apnea. It doesn't matter how beautiful your smile is if you are getting terrible sleep. Fortunately, treating sleep apnea with a simple dental device or sleep breathing machine can immediately improve health, increase job performance, and even save marriages.

4 - Clenching and grinding your teeth is a subtle but devastating problem. Most people are not even aware that they do it. Our teeth are designed to only touch each other only when we chew, swallow, or speak. When teeth contact each other outside those times it can cause chipped and broken teeth, wearing down the teeth, enlarged or oversized chewing muscles, and chronic headaches. Over time the teeth will wear down somewhat but having flattened molars or wear on the front teeth is a sign of something going wrong. I have seen patients who literally wore their teeth down to the gums, like tree stumps in a cleared forest. That is not healthy! It is important to resolve clenching and grinding issues before you get cosmetic dental work--otherwise you'll just grind away your investment! Tooth enamel is the hardest substance in the body. If you have worn down the enamel on your teeth you can definitely chip or break porcelain crowns and veneers.

5 - Our teeth need to do the job of chewing. There are two types of teeth in our mouth, those designed for cutting food (incisors) and those designed for crushing food (molars). When the back teeth are gone the front teeth take on the additional job of crushing the food. This causes the front teeth to chip, break and wear down. Sometimes patients come to me wanting to put veneers on their front teeth, but they don't want to do anything about replacing the missing or broken back teeth necessary to support their chewing. I point out that their front teeth need cosmetic work *because* of the lack of back teeth support. Fixing the teeth that *don't* show when we smile (as well as the teeth that do show) is critical to building a beautiful, lasting smile.

5 – WHAT IS THE BEST SOLUTION?

What is the best way to fix your teeth? The best solution is the one that fits into your life, and that is different for every patient. The treatment you choose must fit into your life 1 - financially, 2 - logistically, and 3 - emotionally.

1 - No matter how badly you want veneers, if buying them puts you in a hard place financially--then veneers don't fit into your life right now.

2 - Some dental treatments require repeated visits over an extended period of time (for example, orthodontics). If you travel a lot or you're moving, the logistics of cosmetic care needs to be planned for.

3 - Some patients who have the time and money to change their smile realize that they don't have the mental or emotional bandwidth to move forward right now. When you select the best cosmetic dental treatment, consider what will *look* best, and what will *work* best for you right now.

As a dentist I have two jobs: make my patients happy and make my patients healthy. I advocate for conservative dental care. In many situations there are multiple options that will produce the same beautiful result. In such cases I always favor the more natural, conservative option. For example, if your teeth are crooked and yellow you could get veneers to cover the teeth, or you could whiten and orthodontically move them to an equally beautiful smile. Veneers are the faster method, but moving your natural teeth is more conservative. Either way, it is most important to consider the overall picture of your life and choose which dental treatment is best for you now.

Stephanie's Story

Stephanie is an actress who lives in L.A. While staying at her vacation home at Lake Tahoe one of her molar crowns came off. She came to me for help to put it back on, and while doing so I noticed significant wear on all of her teeth. We talked about the likely causes of the damage, the long-term consequences, and the benefits of a smile makeover to improve her chewing and enhance her smile.

We did a temporary mockup of what her new smile could look like and she excitedly wore it home on a "test drive" to see what her boyfriend thought. He loved her new smile. However, when she texted a photo to her agent to get his opinion, he raised valid concerns. He pointed out that she was on vacation between shooting seasons of an Amazon series where her character needed to maintain a consistent appearance from season to season. Additionally, she was known in the film industry as a specific type of character and changing her smile could unintentionally place her into a different category of roles. From a career perspective he did not recommend making a major cosmetic change for several years, no matter how much she loved the new look. After considering this she decided that the solution that fit into her life best was to do the work necessary to minimize further wear and have a healthy mouth without making any major cosmetic changes.

Shane Sykes, DMD

6 – ENGINEERING A PERFECT SMILE

There are basic principles of esthetic smiles that dentists follow when building a smile. They are rules of symmetry, form, proportion and size. By following these rules, we get a predictably beautiful smile. You don't need to understand these rules but becoming familiar with them may help you make informed decisions about your new smile.

Humans have three basic types of smiles:
1. Mona Lisa smile,
2. Social smile,
3. Spontaneous smile.

The Mona Lisa smile is the type of closed lip smile we might use to greet a stranger in an elevator. It doesn't show any teeth. The social smile is your carefully practiced and excessively posted selfie smile! A spontaneous smile reveals your true personality and is the target for cosmetic dentistry. If you want to get scientific and geek out on dental details, read on! The rest of this chapter dives into the specific parameters of designing a perfect smile. Feel free to skip ahead if I bore you!

Shane Sykes, DMD

The Ten Commandments of Smile Design[13]:

1.   Starting Point: Everything in the smile should be based upon the *two central incisors* in their proper position relative to the lips and face.

The rest of the teeth should follow an upward curve that traces the lower lip. The central incisors and canines should sit on this line, while the lateral incisors should sit 0.5 - 1.5 mm above it (higher for women, lower for men).

2.   Central Incisors: The upper central incisors should be 75 - 85% as wide as they are tall.

They should be as symmetrical as possible, with the biting edge symmetry being the most critical.

3.   Proportion: There should be a relative size change between the teeth.

The "golden ratio" states that, when viewed from the front, the central incisor should be 1.6x the width of the lateral incisor and the canine should be 0.6x the width of the lateral incisor.

4.   Spaces: Spaces between the teeth, called diastemas, should generally be avoided.

5.   Gingival Margins: The gumline, or gingival margin, of the central incisors should be equal with or slightly below the canines.

The gingival margin of the lateral incisors should be slightly below the central incisors.

Left/right symmetry is crucial.

6.   Gingival Display: There should be less than 3mm of gingiva showing in the smile.

It is acceptable to not have any gums showing. (This rule is largely controlled by genetics.)

7.   Buccal Corridor: The buccal corridor is the space between the sides of the back teeth and the

corner of the lips. The space here should be "middle of the road."

A narrow upper jaw will leave too much space (making the jaw look too small for the face), and a wide upper jaw results in a smile that is "all teeth."

8. Midline and Angulation: The midline between the teeth should be vertical and in the middle of the face.

The angulation of all the teeth should converge toward the belly button.

9. Color and Shape: White teeth with some color closer to the gums are highly desirable. (However, I recommend using your eyes as a guide--if your teeth are whiter than the whites of your eyes people tend to look at your teeth instead of looking at your eyes when you talk.)

Black spaces between the teeth and gums should be avoided.

The corners of the incisal edge should be slightly rounded.

10. Lips: Voluminous lips are the current standard of beauty.

The lips should have adequate support by the teeth and gums.

Markisha's Story

Markisha came to me complaining about how she hated her teeth because "they're yellow like dirty dishwater and they have a gap so big you can drive a truck through it." And she was right! Her teeth were artistically colorful, and she had a gap between her two front teeth that was almost wide enough to fit an extra tooth in. She was insistent that she wanted veneers on the two front teeth to fix both problems. Unfortunately, her teeth were already short, and placing veneers over the two front teeth to close the space would make them much wider than they were tall. I explained the ten commandments of perfect smiles and how I felt she would benefit from orthodontically closing the space rather than covering it with veneers, but she seemed unconvinced. In an effort to show her how terrible it would look, I offered her a quick "test drive" to see what wide veneers would look like. I simply added some white filling material on her teeth to close the gap, then handed her the mirror. We were both shocked at how it improved her smile, even though it grossly violated the ten commandments. In the end she chose invisible braces to close the gaps, along with contouring her gums to create a gorgeous smile. Not only did that allow us to achieve a more pleasing result, it was also the least invasive treatment option.

7 – HOW MUCH WILL THIS COST?

Dentistry is famous for being expensive. There's no denying it, you can invest a lot of money in improving your smile, plus, it's an investment that is usually made solely on trust because you cannot see the end product before you make the investment! It's like buying a new car without ever sitting inside it first.

What patients often overlook is the custom nature of dental work and the harsh conditions it must survive. All that customization and high-quality workmanship takes money to create. Think of it this way: You can buy the latest and greatest iPhone for about the same cost as a porcelain veneer. Both of them are at the cutting edge of what technology can provide, and both are beautiful and functional. Both also require ongoing investment of time and money, (through charging and cellular plans or through daily hygiene and dental cleanings.) However, your phone isn't the first thing you show to every person you meet. You don't use your glass-faced phone to crush solid ice one moment then bite into sizzling hot pizza the next. You don't soak your fancy iPhone in acidic soda or bathe it in corrosive coffee and smoke. You don't use a delicate phone to tear open packages or let bacterial plaque grow all over it. You don't use a phone as a tool to crush or bend things, and you don't clench or grind on it when you're stressed or sleeping. And while your iPhone was mass produced in a factory in China--yes, yes, we all know it was "Designed in California"--your porcelain veneers were delicately hand crafted by a team of master artists specifically to complement your skin, your eyes, and your personality.

Everything about dentistry is customized. So instead of comparing an investment in improving your smile to buying a *normal* car, compare it to hiring someone to build a completely *custom* vehicle designed entirely around you. Think of it like getting a custom Rolls Royce built just for you by Leonardo da Vinci!

Because the cost of dental treatment varies tremendously depending on specific treatment needs, in this book I have provided a generic price range for procedures. This price guide is intended to help you get an idea of how two similar options *compare* financially--not to tell you that you can get your smile fixed for a *specific* amount.

If you are fortunate enough to have dental insurance, you have a head start financially! Although most dental benefit plans do not provide coverage for elective cosmetic treatment or complex restorative care, they will help you have a healthy foundation upon which to build your beautiful new smile.

The last area of cost to consider is *opportunity cost*. Unfortunately, there is a sad but very real cost to having a bad smile. Our physical appearance influences how trustworthy and competent we appear to others. People around you may see a glaring problem in your smile, but they may be too timid to tell you to your face that you need to get your smile fixed. If there is something in your smile that detracts from your appearance it could literally be costing you money to *not* get it fixed.

Jared's Story

Several years ago, Jared came to me for help. He explained that twenty years ago his left front tooth was knocked out in an accident on a construction site. Jared and his wife were struggling newlyweds at the time and he didn't have the money to get it fixed, so he left the hole in his smile. Over the following years he worked hard and was promoted within the company. As their financial situation improved, his wife pleaded with him to get his tooth fixed so she wouldn't be embarrassed going out with him. Jared didn't see any value in it and ignored her pleading. Jared was a smart and dedicated employee, but he plateaued in his construction career well below where he thought he should.

Eventually he became frustrated and finally approached his boss, the owner of the custom home building company, and asked why he was repeatedly passed over for promotions.

His boss grimaced, took a deep breath, then said "Jared, you are the best man we have for that job. I'd love to have you lead our customer relations team, but you don't fit the image we represent to our clients. I can't give you the promotion you deserve while you have a big hole in your smile."

(continued on next page)

Jared's Story - continued

Four days later Jared was in my office looking for a solution, and four weeks later he was in his new position, connecting with wealthy clients planning their dream homes. The cost to fix Jared's smile pales in comparison to the cost of missed opportunities to grow in his profession

Part Two

Smile Solutions

Shane Sykes, DMD

8 – SHORT-TERM SOLUTIONS

The easiest and fastest way to replace missing teeth is with what we call an interim partial denture, often called a "flipper." This is like a retainer that has teeth on it. A flipper can be used to replace a single tooth or multiple teeth. Another option is a product called a "Snap-on Smile." This is a device that covers all your existing teeth and allows us to fabricate a new smile that represents the color and shape you want in your new teeth. The advantages of these short-term solutions are that they are very quick to fabricate (sometimes we can even make them the same day), they are fairly low cost, and they can look quite good. Although short term solutions are low cost (compared to permanent cosmetic solutions), they suffer from poor durability--they are *short term* solutions. Many temporary cosmetic solutions are not designed to be used for eating, only for appearance.

Cost: The cost for a short-term device ranges from $500 to $2000.

Time: The time required to fabricate the device is usually just a few days.

Risks: The primary risk in a short-term solution often lies in the incomplete nature of the treatment. Sometimes people want to use these devices in place of comprehensive care and unfortunately only receive a superficial exam. This leaves undiagnosed conditions that could affect your health and well-being. Furthermore, because the appliances are relatively weak there's a potential for them to break at the most inconvenient moment.

Maintenance: As with all removable devices, keeping temporary appliances clean is critical to extending their useful life and keeping them looking beautiful. An additional area of maintenance that many people do not consider is storage. Pets love to eat these things and I have replaced many, many devices because they were left on the counter and then chewed up by a dog!

Life expectancy: With appropriate wear and care a temporary appliance should be able to last up to six months. However, they can break if you use them for eating and their lifespan will depend largely upon how carefully you treat them.

Replacement options: Temporary appliances should be replaced with a permanent partial, porcelain veneers, a bridge or dental implants.

David's Story

David came to my office in a moment of crisis. He is a competitive Strong Man and was preparing for an important event. In training that morning he was lifting a massive 250-pound Atlas Stone onto a platform when it rolled backwards and hit him in the face, breaking one of his front teeth irreparably. He didn't have time before the event to replace the tooth with a dental implant, but he knew that was the long-term solution he wanted. We were able to quickly make him a flipper to replace the missing tooth so that he could go to his competition with confidence. Later he returned to replace the tooth with an implant.

Shane Sykes, DMD

9 – TEETH WHITENING

No doubt about it the best way you can enhance your smile is to simply *use it!* No matter what your smile looks like, if you will smile with genuine joy the beauty of your smile will come out and people will appreciate it. The most cost-effective and impactful way to enhance that natural smile is to whiten your teeth. Excuse me as I climb on my soapbox for a moment: we commonly use the word "bleaching" to refer to improving the whiteness of our teeth. I want to be very clear about this: DO NOT PUT BLEACH ON YOUR TEETH!!! Putting bleach in your mouth could result in very bad consequences! However, there are many whitening materials that can be used with great safety. Dismount soapbox.

Many people ask me if whitening damages their teeth, and that depends upon what whitening materials you are using. Whitening materials are very unstable, so many manufacturers add acids to extend the shelf-life. Using an acidic product on your tooth can damage tooth enamel if used excessively or improperly. The best whitening materials are a neutral pH or have additional beneficial ingredients like fluoride, desensitizers and remineralizing agents in them so that your teeth will actually be more healthy and cavity resistant after whitening than before.

All products that whiten teeth effectively have some form of peroxide in them. Whether it is Crest White Strips from the grocery store or Zoom whitening done in the dental office, effective whitening products all use the same basic chemistry.

DIY Whitening: Most Do-It-Yourself tooth whitening will be useless at best and harmful at worst. There are many over the counter and home remedies that sort-of work, but there are many more that are just a waste of money. There are some products, like toothpastes and rinses, that claim to whiten teeth with no effect. Others claim to whiten teeth but do so by removing surface stains with harsh abrasives that can damage your teeth. There are a few at-home remedies that can provide a tiny bit of whitening through acids applied to the tooth, for example mashed strawberries can provide some whitening benefit.

The next step above homemade remedies is the peroxide-based whitening products available at the grocery store. These can be effective and give a good result if they are applied properly to the teeth. In my experience mouthwashes that claim to whiten the teeth are not a high enough peroxide concentration or do not stay in contact with the teeth anywhere near long enough to produce any noticeable whitening in a reasonable time period.

Products like Crest White Strips can be very effective when used properly. If you use this type of product, please be aware that you can injure your gums if you apply the whitening strip in a way that it touches your gums. Many of these types of products only cover the front six teeth, so you can end up with a funny-looking smile because the back teeth do not get whitened like the front teeth. And unless you are very meticulous in scalloping the strips into the curves between the teeth you may end up with dark or colored stripes in between your teeth.

To get the best results in whitening your teeth I highly recommend professional whitening. There are two options for professional whitening: at-home and in-office.

Professional At-Home Whitening: At-home whitening is the staple of professional whitening, and I have never had a patient who couldn't get satisfactory results with the right techniques of at-home whitening. When my mother was about 65 years old she was interested in whitening her teeth so I made her some at-home trays. She was able to whiten from the darkest color on the whitening scale to the lightest color in six months. (Most people notice a similarly dramatic change in just weeks, not months, so perhaps it took that long to achieve those results because I was giving her our leftover, expired whitening materials!)

One of the concerns some patients experience with whitening is tooth sensitivity. This is caused by "too much, too fast," and can be avoided by managing how long you wear the trays in your mouth, how frequently you wear the trays, and the concentration of the whitening gel you use. With the right products and techniques anyone can whiten their teeth without experiencing unmanageable sensitivity.

In-Office Whitening: The fastest way to get white teeth is in-office whitening. Unfortunately, this is an area where many people can be swindled. The key ingredient of in-office whitening is still peroxide, but there are also many systems designed to excite or wow patients with fancy whitening lights or lasers or gadgets. There is little to no research that any of these devices actually do anything--they just provide a way for your dentist to look fancy and charge you more while the in-office peroxide does it's work.

The advantage of in-office whitening is that it will give you noticeable results after just one treatment. It is followed up with custom at-home whitening for continued improvement in color. In-office whitening is particularly popular among my patients who are rushing to get ready for a wedding, a reunion, or family photos.

Internal Whitening: Lastly, when you have a single tooth that has died and turned dark and will not respond to normal whitening, we can whiten the tooth from the inside-out. This is accomplished by making a special space inside the tooth to hold the whitening material. In most cases the dark tooth has already had a root canal treatment, or it needs to have one. Internal whitening works very well, especially when used in conjunction with professional whitening of the other teeth.

Regardless of what method you choose to whiten your teeth, whitening provides more "bang for your buck" in improving your smile than any other cosmetic procedure. I use it as the starting point for all other cosmetic work. The color in your teeth will rebound just a little and stabilize during the two weeks after you whiten, and a freshly whitened tooth does not bond to dental composites as strongly as normal until two weeks after whitening. Be aware that you need to wait two weeks after whitening to do other cosmetic work

My team and I donate 100% of the proceeds from our whitening procedures to the Smiles For Life Children's Foundation. Our dental supplier donates the materials, we donate our time, and our patients make a donation to the charity. Over the past 20 years my colleagues and I have raised over $40,000,000 for charity through whitening. You can learn more and get involved with this great work at www.SmilesForLife.org. *Whiten your smile and help a child!*

Cost: While you can waste as much money as you want on DIY whitening, professional whitening ranges from $200 to $800, with specialized whitening for complex coloring costing up to $1,500.

Time: In-office whitening produces significant results after one visit. Professional at-home whitening usually takes two to three weeks for maximum results.

Risks: Poorly managed whitening can cause temporary tooth sensitivity and gum irritation. Teeth are more sensitive to stain during the whitening process, so while whitening I recommend you avoid smoking or eating and drinking anything that would stain a white t-shirt.

Maintenance: Your teeth gradually discolor after whitening. Most people find that a simple touch-up whitening every 12 months keeps them sparkling white. If you have professional at-home trays you can also touch-up with one or two treatments before photos or a special event. Storing your whitening gel in the fridge will extend its shelf life.

Life Expectancy: Whitening doesn't last forever, but it can be done at any age!

Replacement Options: If whitening doesn't get you the results you want, porcelain veneers are the best alternative.

Allison's Story

Allison was a busy mother of three and was quite a social butterfly. Her own parents had taken great care of her and she had regular dental visits as a child and braces as a teenager, so she had perfectly straight and healthy teeth. Unfortunately, when she was quite young she was treated with Tetracycline, an antibiotic that frequently causes dark brown horizontal lines in developing teeth. So although she had straight teeth, they weren't the pearly whites she wanted. She had tried Crest whitestrips but just ended up burning her gums. To make matters worse, she already had sensitive teeth! Through a special combination of desensitizing medications, in-office treatments and at-home trays Allison was able to get a dazzling white smile. She was delighted that she finally had a smile that matched her bright and bubbly personality, and one that she didn't feel she wanted to hide every time she laughed.

10 – GUM TREATMENTS

Like beautiful architecture requires a good foundation, a beautiful smile must have healthy gums (called gingiva) as a foundation. There are a number of gum treatments that can improve your smile, ranging from improving the health of your gums to changing the shape of your gums.

Gingivitis and gum disease (Periodontitis) affect 80% of all adults in the USA. This often starts as puffy, swollen, and red gums around the teeth that bleed when you brush or floss. Healthy gums do not bleed, so if your gums bleed during routine hygiene it may be a sign of gingivitis or an infection. Improving your gum health will improve the appearance of the teeth and may have a dramatic effect on your overall appearance.

Bacteria hiding in the mouth cause halitosis (AKA bad breath!). Nearly everyone with a gum infection has bad breath. Fortunately, this is easily resolved when the gums become healthy.

One of the reasons someone may want to change their smile is to improve their romantic life. Since gum disease, bad breath, and cavities are a bacterial infection they can be transmitted by kissing. I like to tease my patients by telling them that once they've treated infections and they get a clean bill of health I'll give them a badge stating that they are "Certified Kissable."

Once the gums are healthy, another gum treatment we can explore is adjusting the *shape* of your gums. Some patients have gum recession that exposes the yellow roots of the teeth. This makes the teeth look strangely long and can also cause black empty triangles to appear between the teeth along the gumline. Gum grafting is a procedure to cover the roots of the teeth and regrow the gums. It is not a particularly pleasant or predictable treatment, but new technology and techniques are continually improving.

The opposite of gum recession is a mouth that shows too much gum when you smile. If your gums cover too much of your teeth the teeth look short and square. This can be quickly solved by contouring the gums to remove the excess tissue. Gum contouring is one of my favorite procedures because it's fast and simple, yet it produces profound results. It is a subtle change--people will look twice at your smile and say "Wow, you look great. Something's different but I can't tell what." Usually we do laser gum contouring with little or no anesthetic and the results are instant. Sometimes only excess gum tissue needs to be removed, other times there is excess bone around the teeth that also needs to be removed. Second to whitening, I think gum contouring provides the greatest value for your investment in improving your smile. When I do other cosmetic procedures like veneers, I almost always do gum contouring too.

Cost: The cost of gum treatment varies widely depending upon the severity of infection and the response of your immune system. It can range from one hundred dollars to thousands of dollars. Similarly, the cost of grafting or gum contouring will vary depending upon where you are starting but can range from $200 to $2,000.

Time: Gum contouring can be accomplished in a single visit. Gum therapy to treat serious infections requires multiple visits spread over about six weeks.

Risks: There are virtually no risks to getting healthy gums. The greatest risk is in *not* treating unhealthy gums, since this can actually cause you to have a heart attack or stroke!

Maintenance: Sometimes the gums grow back years after gum contouring, which requires a minor touch-up. Patients with gum infections need to see the dental hygienist every 3-4 months to keep their gums healthy.

Life Expectancy: Treating gum disease will literally increase your life expectancy. People with unhealthy gums have a 12-20% higher risk of premature death[14].

Replacement options: If the gums are not healthy and teeth are lost, the teeth can be replaced with bridges, implants or dentures.

Sandy's Story

Sandy felt like she had a healthy mouth, but she wanted to improve the appearance of her smile. She had dark, discolored teeth that were crowded and "look like the Grinch"--her words, not mine! As we evaluated Sandy's oral health together, she was shocked to discover that she had a severe gum infection. Gum disease, like diabetes and heart disease, is usually painless and has no symptoms (except for bad breath) until it is in its most severe stages. Sandy had deep pockets harboring toxic bacterial plaque that was eating away the bone supporting her teeth. The bacteria were also leaking into her bloodstream and putting her at higher risk for a heart attack or a stroke. Unfortunately, several of her teeth were so severely infected they were beyond repair and had to be removed. We treated the remaining teeth and gums to get them healthy and white before we replaced her missing teeth. This improved her smile dramatically. She was thrilled! When I saw her for routine follow-up six months later, I was shocked at how her overall appearance had improved. Sandy and I looked at her pre-treatment photos and we realized that previously she had a waxen, green, sickly tone to her complexion. Now her skin was clear, firm, and lustrous. Getting rid of her gum infection had made her more healthy, vibrant and confident. In addition to the cosmetic benefits of her smile makeover, she now had the confidence and motivation to quit smoking--further improving her overall health!

11 -- ORTHODONTICS

Straightening your teeth is a natural and healthy way to improve your smile. Thanks to modern technology there are many different options to straighten your teeth that do not require the ugly metal braces you may have been teased about as a child. Orthodontic treatment can be used to move a few teeth into a more ideal position, used as part of a comprehensive plan, or used as a standalone solution to completely straighten your smile. There are three types of braces available today: traditional braces, invisible aligners, and lingual braces.

Traditional braces: The tried-and-true method for straightening teeth is the same braces that have been used for decades, but with many modern advancements. In addition to traditional metal brackets, now we have white and clear brackets used with metal wires to straighten the teeth more stealthily and inconspicuously. Although there are other options that are less visible, in some cases these alternatives can't match the ideal results we will get with traditional braces. Traditional braces are fantastic because they require no effort from you, the patient; they just do their work 24/7. One of the disadvantages of traditional braces is the difficulty of keeping them clean. It requires dedication and discipline to properly clean around the braces in order to keep the gums healthy and avoid developing cavities during orthodontic treatment.

Invisible aligners: Thanks to companies like Invisalign, straightening teeth has never been easier or more cosmetic. Clear aligners are transparent plastic trays that fit perfectly over your teeth. You wear them all day and all night, except while eating. You wear each aligner for one to two weeks, then throw that tray away and wear the next aligner tray (which is shaped slightly differently than the previous tray). As you progress through the series of aligners the teeth gradually move toward the perfect position. Aligners are super convenient and easy to use, plus you can take the aligners out to eat and clean your teeth -- avoiding the hassles of traditional braces! The benefit of clear aligners is that they are practically invisible, and they are removable to clean your teeth. The disadvantage of clear aligners is that because they are removable, it requires discipline and willpower to wear them. If they are not in your mouth, they will not move your teeth. You can't take a vacation from wearing your aligners. The best thing about Invisalign is that it's removable, the worst thing about Invisalign is that it's... removable!

There are several less reputable aligner companies that will scan your teeth at a booth in a mall or send you supplies to make impressions of your teeth at home. Then they mail you aligners to treat yourself at home. These companies use basically the same technology we use in the dental office, but I have serious concerns about this method of treatment. While these companies usually have a dentist on staff and claim that your case is "reviewed and approved" by a licensed dentist, they do not screen for gum disease or other dental complications. If you have a gum infection or other problems, it is possible to move your teeth right out of the jaw! I do not recommend do-it-yourself aligners unless you have consulted with your dentist.

Lingual braces: The ultimate invisible teeth-straightening system is braces that are glued to the tongue-side of your teeth. Like the dark side of the moon, no one will ever see the brackets on the back side of your teeth! Using a 3D camera, we can scan your jaws, then digitally plan and robotically fabricate custom wires to move your teeth.

At first the brackets may bother your tongue, but tongues are pretty adept at learning how to avoid being irritated by the braces. Many patients prefer lingual braces over traditional braces for the improved comfort as well as cosmetics. They are also easier to keep clean than traditional braces.

Retainers: Yes, you need retainers. Regardless of which orthodontic treatment you choose, once your teeth have moved you will need to wear retainers to "retain" your teeth in their new alignment for as long as you want your teeth to stay straight.

There are two different styles of retainers: permanent and removable. Permanent retainers are glued to the tongue side of the teeth and thoughtlessly keep the teeth in their straight position. Permanent retainers have the advantage of being permanent -- you don't need to remember to put retainers in at night -- but they do require significantly more time and attention to floss and clean.

Removable retainers can be either acrylic with a wire or clear aligner type retainers. These must be worn every night for as long as you want your teeth to stay straight. The advantage of removable retainers is that they are removable! That makes your teeth easy to clean. The disadvantage of removable retainers is that they are removable. They can get lazily forgotten. Or lost. Or broken. Or thrown away. Or dropped in the sink disposal grinder. Or eaten by your dog. Yes, I've made new retainers for all those reasons and more!

Cost: You can expect to spend $2,000 - $8,000 on orthodontic treatment, depending upon the length of treatment and the type of braces.

Time: Minor straightening can be as short as three months, while complex straightening may take up to two years.

Risks: Some of the risks of orthodontic treatment are:

- Trauma to the lips and tongue,
- Cavities,
- Gum irritation due to a lack of hygiene,
- Bone loss around the teeth if the gums are not kept healthy,
- In rare cases the roots of the teeth can shrink when the teeth are moved orthodontically.

Maintenance: In addition to meticulous brushing and flossing, during orthodontic treatment it is essential to have regular dental cleanings to keep your teeth and gums healthy. Following treatment, you must wear retainers nightly for long as you want your teeth to stay straight!

Life expectancy: Orthodontic treatment will give you a beautiful smile that will last the rest of your life -- if you wear your retainers!

Alternative options: Veneers are a common and popular way to get the same cosmetic results in a shorter time than orthodontics requires.

Millie's Story

Millie was a lively, friendly 80-year-old woman who had been coming to our practice for many years. During a routine check-up I sat back and asked her "Millie, we've been seeing you for many years and your teeth have always been healthy, but I want to check in and see if there's anything you would like to change about your smile."

She started to say something, hesitated, then timidly started to point to her teeth before saying "I wondered... never mind."

I encouraged her to go on and she pointed to one of her front teeth that stuck out in front of her other teeth. With some emotion she said "I've always hated this tooth and the way it sticks out. Is there anything you can do about that?"

Within the hour she had started orthodontic treatment and six months later she had the smile that she had wanted all her life! You're never too old to have the smile you deserve.

Shane Sykes, DMD

12 -- ENAMELOPLASTY

Chapters 8-11 have discussed *non-invasive* care. We are not removing or reshaping the teeth, just changing the position, color or gums. Chapters 12-20 will address *invasive* treatments. The most simple and conservative invasive treatment we can provide is enameloplasty -- what I sometimes refer to as "a manicure for your smile." This involves polishing away some of the natural tooth material to create a better shape or contour. Even a very subtle change in the shape of a tooth can make a dramatic difference in the way it looks and is far more conservative than most alternatives.

Enameloplasty can: make slightly crooked teeth appear straight; even out the biting edges of teeth; or round and soften the corners of square teeth to make them more pleasing. I never need to use anesthetic for patients when doing enameloplasty, because if we are polishing deep enough that it causes discomfort then enameloplasty alone is not the right solution. In that case we would protect the sensitive areas of the tooth with a different solution.

I usually do a little bit of enameloplasty on most cosmetic patients, especially to put the finishing touch on a beautiful smile after Invisalign treatment.

Cost: Reshaping teeth can cost from $50 to $250, depending on the number of teeth involved.

Time: The procedure is completed in a single visit.

Risks: Overly aggressive enameloplasty may cause tooth sensitivity.

Maintenance: Nothing beyond routine dental care is required.

Life expectancy: Enameloplasty will not affect the life expectancy of your teeth.

Alternative options: Veneers are a great alternative if treatment beyond enameloplasty is required.

Brenda's Story

I first met Brenda as a new patient coming into our office for routine care. She had beautiful white teeth and a gorgeous smile, but I noticed that one of her front teeth was just a tiny bit longer than the other. I was hesitant to point it out because I didn't want it to bother her, but I knew that I could provide a solution to fix it that would be minimally invasive and instantaneous. I timidly asked if there's anything she wanted to change about her smile and she said no, she didn't think there was anything to change. I pointed out the discrepancy between the two front teeth and asked if she had noticed how one tooth was longer than the other. She mentioned that she had noticed it but didn't want to go through the pain and expense of braces to change it so she just learned to accept it. I offered to polish the long tooth just a little bit shorter to match the other and see how she liked it. Thirty seconds later the two teeth were even, and she was absolutely thrilled with the result!

12 -- BONDING

Bonding is another conservative way to improve the appearance of misshapen teeth. I'm not talking about sitting around a campfire singing Kumbaya, I'm talking about cosmetic tooth bonding. This process uses white filling material bonded to the surface of the tooth to add shape and structure. Bonding can also cover discoloration and stains. Bonding can be accomplished in a single visit at a lower cost than many other alternatives. Enameloplasty is almost always done in conjunction with bonding. One great advantage of bonding is that in most cases it is completely reversible. Simply polishing away the filling material will reveal the original tooth underneath.

Bonding can be done on a single tooth or on the entire smile. It is a great solution in trauma cases, for example when a front tooth has broken from a bicycle crash. Bonding is also useful in kids and teens, where the teeth and gums are still maturing so we would not want to do porcelain veneers.

Cost: Bonding is usually charged per tooth, with a fee that ranges from $300 to $1,000 per tooth, depending on the complexity.

Time: Most bonding can be done instantly with a few follow-up visits for refinement.

Risks: Over time the bonding material will begin to discolor. The bonding material can fracture or get cavities around it. Poorly finished bonding can result in gum irritation.

Maintenance: Bonding does not require any special maintenance beyond what you already do for your natural teeth. However, bonding material does not change color with teeth whitening, so it is important to make sure you are happy with the color of your natural teeth before bonding.

Life expectancy: With routine care you can expect your bonding to last for 10 years before you start to notice staining or a rough surface. I have seen cases where bonding lasted for twenty years before it became undesirable.

Replacement Options: When bonding has served its useful life, it can simply be polished away or it can be replaced with new bonding or with porcelain veneers for a more long-lasting solution.

Vanessa's Story

Vanessa was referred to me by one of her friends for whom I had recently treated with veneers. Vanessa was self-conscious of the gap between her two front teeth. She was tired of hiding her smile and wondered if veneers would work for her too. Vanessa's teeth were a beautiful shape and color, so I proposed bonding as a simpler solution rather than veneers.

Vanessa agreed, and without the need for anesthetic or drilling on her teeth, I placed bonding material on her teeth and closed the gap. She was thrilled that it was so fast and easy. When I handed her the mirror to see her new smile she started giggling like a child. She hugged every person in the office before she left and seemed to float on a cloud as she left.

You can imagine my surprise two weeks later when she came into the office in tears. I thought something had gone wrong and her beautiful new teeth had broken. I was relieved when she smiled and saw her bonding still intact. Then she explained to me that although she loved the way her new teeth looked, she felt that it just wasn't her. She didn't recognize the woman staring back in the mirror and she felt like she had lost part of her identity. Until the gap between her two front teeth was gone, she didn't realize it was a special part of her personality. She now recognized that her desire to eliminate the gap was really just wanting to be like other people rather than being true to herself. She tearfully asked what we could do to get her original smile back. She was flooded with relief when I explained that we could simply polish away the material we bonded on and she would be back to her familiar smile. After a few minutes of polishing to reveal her natural teeth again, she once more gave us all hugs and left on cloud nine, confident in who she was and her intrinsic beauty and worth.

14 – REPLACING OLD FILLINGS

Compared to years past, today's dental materials are both attractive and durable. Unfortunately, older materials were either attractive OR durable, and dentists leaned heavily toward durable materials at the expense of appearance. Because of this many people have old white fillings that aren't white anymore, or visible black metal fillings on their back teeth.

I'm not going to address the highly contentious issue of Mercury-Amalgam fillings other than to say that the first day I had my own practice was the *last* day I placed a mercury filling. Old black fillings can be easily and safely replaced with white fillings. I don't encourage patients to replace cavity-free metal fillings, but I am happy to replace them when patients request it for cosmetic or holistic purposes.

When old metal fillings begin to break down or get cavities (which happens to *every* type of filling eventually) I recommend replacing them with white composite fillings. As metal fillings age they corrode and turn black. The corrosion can leach into the tooth and turn the entire tooth black. If the black stain is significant the tooth may need a crown or veneer to hide the discoloration.

Over time white fillings and bonding will begin to discolor. Sometimes we can polish them to remove surface stains and extend their useful life, but if the stain is deep in the material the filling will need to be replaced.

Cost: Replacing fillings will cost $200-$500 per tooth, depending on the size of the filling.

Time: Single or multiple replacement fillings can be completed in a single visit.

Risks: Every time we replace a filling the new filling is slightly larger. Excessively large fillings weaken teeth and should be replaced with crowns.

Maintenance: Nothing beyond routine dental care is required.

Life expectancy: Fillings are expected to last 7-10 years.

Replacement options: Crowns and veneers are a great alternative if treatment beyond replacement fillings is required.

My Own Story

Although I am a dentist now and understand the importance of brushing my teeth, as a child I was not so diligent, and I ended up with several cavities that were treated with metal fillings. As I became educated in dentistry, I decided that eventually I would replace my metal fillings with white composite, but only as they needed it due to deterioration. However, one evening I photobombed my son by sneaking up behind him and opening my mouth wide, pretending to bite off his ear. The resulting photo was quite comical, but I was horrified at the sight of a big black filling glistening on my lower molar. It was the only thing I could focus on in the photo! I immediately called my partner and asked him to stay late after work the next day to replace all my black fillings. I didn't want an ugly tooth to ruin my photobombing ever again!

Shane Sykes, DMD

15 – VENEERS AND CROWNS

When most people think about cosmetic dentistry, they think about porcelain veneers. Modern porcelain is absolutely beautiful and can look every bit as life-like as completely natural teeth. Porcelain is used to create the Hollywood smile in so many of today's celebrities. While there are many different variations of "fixed prosthetics" (laminate porcelain veneer, inlay, onlay, ¾ crown, reverse ¾ crown,....) I will refer to them all as veneers and crowns. A crown is used to cover part or all of the tooth, like how a football helmet protects your head. A veneer is a thin sheet of porcelain that is placed over the surface of the tooth, like a press-on fingernail. Both can deliver gorgeous results and are frequently used together in cosmetic makeovers. I decide if I'll use a crown or a veneer based on the strength and shape of the underlying tooth. For simplicity I will treat them interchangeably here, because they are made from the same materials.

Crowns can be made from a number of different materials, and new products continue to emerge with increasingly better results. Gone are the days when getting a crown meant having a shiny gold tooth or a chalky white tooth with an ugly black line where the metal shows underneath. With metal-free porcelain crowns and veneers there is a trade-off between strength and beauty; and in general, the stronger the material is the less life-like it appears. Choosing the right material is important for both the appearance and the longevity of your new smile.

We make gorgeous crowns right in our office in a single visit. I typically use made-in-office crowns on back teeth to provide maximum durability with great cosmetics. This has the advantage of being fast and convenient without the need for a temporary crown. Same-day crowns have cosmetic limitations, so when seeking ideal cosmetics, I order custom crowns and veneers from a dental laboratory. There artists meticulously sculpt and paint each individual tooth for an exquisite result. Meanwhile, you wear temporary crowns that simulate the shape and appearance of the desired result.

One of the advantages of porcelain veneers and crowns is that they do not change color and darken over time like natural teeth and bonding do. This means that your smile will stay bright and white forever. However, it also means that if you whiten your teeth in the future, your veneers will not change color. Therefore, it is very important that you whiten your natural teeth to a color you are happy with before selecting the final color for your new veneers.

Prepless Veneers: When the teeth are already in a relatively favorable position, we can use prepless veneers to change the color or the shape of the teeth. Placing a thin layer of porcelain over the tooth makes a dramatic cosmetic improvement without changing any of the natural tooth. There are a few well-marketed brands of prepless veneers (Lumineers, Dura-Thin Veneers, Radiant Veneers) that all use the same basic technique. Prepless veneers work well in smiles where few changes are needed. They are applied without any anesthetic because we are not changing the shape of the natural tooth, but I often use enameloplasty in conjunction with prepless veneers. If the tooth is too far out of position or the color change needed is too great, other solutions may work better.

Traditional Veneers/Crowns: When the teeth are misaligned, weakened, or in an unfavorable or unhealthy position, sometimes it is necessary to polish away part of the existing tooth structure so that we can replace it with porcelain. The porcelain can also be used to cover teeth that have discolored due to old fillings, root canals, or internal discoloration.

Cost: Veneers and crowns are generally charged per tooth, with a price of $1,000 - $2,000 each.

Time: Some crowns can be made in a single visit in the dental office, while others are sent to the lab with a turnaround time of three to five weeks.

Risks: While modern porcelain is very strong, it is a glass material and can chip, crack or break. Porcelain crowns and veneers can be compared to porcelain floor tiles. If you pick up a tile off the shelf at Home Depot you can easily break it, but once it is bonded to the floor of the Mercedes Benz showroom you can drive a car on it. But if you drop a hammer on the tile floor it may crack. Similarly, veneers and crowns are tremendously strong but can crack with uneven force. That means no biting your fingernails, opening packages, or bending bobby-pins -- *teeth are not tools!*

As with any invasive treatment on the tooth, there's a risk of nerve irritation.

And there's the possibility that the bond may fail and a veneer or crown could fall off.

Maintenance: Just like your natural teeth, porcelain crowns and veneers require routine maintenance to keep things healthy. Just because the teeth are covered with porcelain does not mean they are immune to cavities! Additionally, in order to protect the porcelain from unhealthy forces from grinding your teeth at night, wearing a night guard is often recommended.

Life expectancy: Well-maintained crowns and veneers can be expected to last 10 to 20 years.

Replacement options: Prepless veneers can be removed without any damage to the underlying teeth and without any replacement. Traditional crowns and veneers that become damaged must be replaced with new crowns or veneers.

Kelly's Story

Kelly came to see me because she was getting married in two months and wanted to make sure that she was healthy and looked her best for her wedding day. During the exam we talked about the discoloration of her front teeth. When she was a child, she got cavities between her two front teeth and they were filled with white filling material. Over the years that filling material had discolored to a band of dark yellow between her two front teeth that she passionately called her "skunk stripe." She was ecstatic when I explained that we could place veneers on her front teeth to replace the ugly fillings and enhance her already beautiful smile. She immediately started whitening her teeth, and three weeks later we made her veneers. When I handed her a mirror so she could look at her new smile she burst into tears. Choked up with sobs of emotion, she simply whispered "Thank you." She explained that she wanted a beautiful wedding but had never dreamed her smile could look this good. Then she broke all the COVID social distancing rules and gave me a big hug and cried on my shoulder. She was a beautiful bride.

Shane Sykes, DMD

16 – ROOT CANAL THERAPY

When I say "root canal" the image in your mind's eye is probably a scene from a horror movie rather than a vision of a beautiful smile. But treating the damaged nerve inside a tooth can produce outstanding cosmetic results. A root canal may be necessary when a tooth is fractured and a nerve is exposed, when a cavity reaches the nerve of the tooth, or when a tooth has abscessed due to trauma. Nerve damage often causes a tooth to turn brown because of bruising and infection inside the tooth.

A root canal treatment is like taking the wick out of a candle. The infected nerve in the tooth is gently removed and the inside of the tooth is disinfected and sealed with a special material. Unfortunately, root canals have a reputation of being unpleasant. But most root canals cause no more discomfort than a routine filling or crown.

A tooth that has had a root canal treatment can become weak. A crown is usually placed to strengthen and support the tooth so that it won't break in the future. Sometimes a dark tooth cannot be whitened with normal techniques. In this situation we may do a root canal and whiten the tooth from the inside. This is one of the healthiest and most dramatic ways to change a smile that has a single dark tooth.

Cost: A root canal costs $1000-2000, depending on the complexity of the root. A crown is also often required at additional expense.

Time: Some root canals can be completed in a single visit. Whitening a tooth from the inside at the roots may take multiple visits.

Risks: Like everything we do in dentistry -- and life -- nothing is 100% successful all of the time. A root canal may fail, become re-infected, or the tooth may crack and break.

Maintenance: A root canal treated tooth requires no special attention beyond routine hygiene.

Life Expectancy: A healthy root canal should last for the rest of your life.

Replacement options: When a root canal treated tooth develops a problem it can be solved by retreatment of the root canal, an apicoectomy (a reverse root canal treatment), or extraction.

Vinny's Story

Vinny had been a patient in my practice for several years. Recently he was in our office for his regular checkup and cleaning. During his exam I noticed that one of his front teeth had turned much darker than the others, so I recommended that we take an x-ray to evaluate the root of the tooth. His x-ray and further testing revealed that the nerve inside the tooth had died and the dead nerve was causing the brown color. Vinny didn't have any pain from the tooth, but he recalled being hit in the face years previously while playing basketball, which is probably what caused the tooth to eventually die years later. I recommended a root canal treatment with internal whitening and Vinny was excited by the possibility of changing the color of that tooth. Together with the internal whitening we also whitened all of his other teeth, resulting in a fabulous smile with minimal treatment.

17 -- BRIDGES

Sometimes teeth are lost due to trauma or infection, and sometimes people are born missing some of their permanent teeth. A dental bridge, technically called a "fixed partial denture," is a wonderful way to replace missing teeth. Bridges rely on your natural teeth on either side of the missing tooth to support a fake tooth, called a "pontic." In certain situations, we are able to build a bridge supported by only one tooth -- with the pontic leveraged in the missing tooth space. We can also make a bridge called a Maryland bridge that is bonded to the surface of the neighboring teeth and does not require covering the entire tooth.

Functionally and cosmetically bridges are very similar to crowns and veneers and are made from the same porcelain materials. Bridges can be used to replace a single tooth or multiple missing teeth. They can be placed on top of dental implants, but we cannot connect a natural tooth and a dental implant together with a bridge. Natural teeth have a shock-absorbing ligament that allows them to move slightly, but implants do not (connecting a tooth and an implant with a bridge may cause one of them to fail). Bridges are usually fabricated in the lab, and in the meantime, you will wear a temporary bridge.

The bone that holds our teeth is a specialized type of bone, and its only job is to hold teeth. Once a tooth is missing the bone around it no longer has a job and it will slowly begin to melt away. This can leave a defect in the bone that may become a problem cosmetically. If the gum and bone underneath the missing tooth are healthy a bridge can look and function just like a natural tooth, but if the bone has resorbed significantly additional gum procedures may be helpful to get rid of the gap under the bridge.

Cost: Bridges are usually charged per tooth involved, at a cost of $1,000 to $2,000 per tooth.

Time: Bridges take 3-6 weeks to fabricate.

Risks: Like crowns, bridges may chip, crack or break, and there is a risk of nerve irritation. When porcelain is bonded to the tooth there's a possibility that the bond could fail, and the bridge could fall off.

Maintenance: In addition to routine dental care, it is necessary to floss *underneath* the bridge with a floss threader -- like putting thread through the eye of a needle.

Life Expectancy: On average you can expect a bridge to last 10 to 20 years, although I have a patient with a perfectly healthy bridge that was placed during World War II!

Replacement Options: When a bridge fails it can be replaced with a new bridge, dental implants, or a removable partial denture.

Misty's Story

Misty was an arrestingly beautiful 30-year-old patient in my practice. She got lucky in the genetic lottery with a tall, slender body and a beautiful face, but her genes were missing the information needed for a full set of permanent teeth. She was missing all four of her lateral incisors (the tooth just to the side of the middle front teeth). As a child she had braces that straightened her teeth where the neighboring teeth had tipped into the missing tooth spaces, and she had been wearing a flipper (a retainer with teeth on it) to replace the missing teeth for the past 20 years. She finally had a great job and she was financially ready to get rid of her flipper. However, Misty was deathly afraid of needles and in the past, she has needed to be put under general anesthesia in a hospital for dental work because she had so much anxiety. So, she was definitely not interested in dental implants, which were my first recommendation for her. Fortunately, with no anesthetic and only minor polishing to correct the contours of her natural teeth, we were able to make four Maryland bridges to replace Misty's missing teeth. The result was gorgeous and natural, and she was so relieved she didn't have to go to the hospital for sedation.

18 – DENTAL IMPLANTS

Often the best solution for missing teeth is replacement with dental implants. Simply put, a dental implant is a titanium root that is placed in the bone, replacing the natural tooth root. The bone grows around the implant and integrates the titanium as a part of your body. Once the implant is integrated, we can place things on top of it, ranging from a single tooth to multiple teeth to removable dentures.

The success of implants depends on your health and habits. In healthy individuals the success rate is very high, while for smokers or people with weak immune systems the success rate is slightly lower. Because infection is the number one cause of tooth loss it is important that your gums are healthy in the area around the implants (to prevent infection or contamination of the new implant).

There are two ways we can place an implant, delayed or immediate. Delayed implants are placed into areas where the tooth has been extracted and the bone has completely healed. In general, this requires six months of healing for the bone to be ready to accept an implant. Then we use a specialized drill to create a hole in the bone into which we place the dental implant. After another six months of healing (a total of twelve months after the extraction) the implant is ready for use.

An immediate implant is when we remove the tooth and immediately place the implant into the hole where the tooth was. This has the advantage of avoiding the healing time that would be required for a delayed implant so you can get to the end result faster. Immediate implants cannot be placed into areas of infection or places where the bone is compromised. In some situations it's possible to place a temporary crown on top of the implant so you can chew on it without waiting for the implant to heal (but this is not done very often because it can put the implant at risk of failing).

Once the implant has healed for six months, we place a piece called an abutment on top of it. The abutment is used to support either a single tooth, a group of teeth in a bridge, or a snap-on denture. Implants can look and function just like natural teeth and caring for them requires the same time and attention as your natural teeth. When there are two implants side by side it is difficult to achieve ideal gum contours between the two implants because the gums respond differently in this situation. Sometimes this can leave a black triangle at the gums between the two teeth, which can be addressed through a few different methods, including using pink porcelain to replace the missing gums.

Dental implants require a minimum of 2mm of bone surrounding the implants on all sides. This means that sometimes there's not enough bone available to place the implant exactly where we want it. Fortunately, today's bone grafting procedures are excellent, and we can usually add bone to the areas we want it to achieve ideal aesthetic and functional results. The most common reason for bone grafting is because there's not enough vertical thickness of bone in the upper jaw, especially around the maxillary sinuses. This can be resolved by adding bone into the sinus through a sinus lift procedure. We also frequently add bone to narrow jaws to make the bone thick enough for an implant.

Cost: Dental implant fees vary widely based upon how many teeth are involved, what parts are used and the health of the bone. A simple single tooth implant will cost $4,000 - $5,000, while a full replacement of teeth including complex grafting can cost up to $30,000 per jaw.

Time: Generally, implants require 6-12 months of total treatment time. The cost of implant treatment is spread out over this time.

Risks: When placing a dental implant, the implant might not properly integrate into the body and may need to be removed. There's also potential for damage to nerves or sinuses. And infections can complicate the surgery.

Maintenance: Dental implants require the same maintenance that natural teeth do.

Life Expectancy: Dental implants are considered to be a lifetime solution.

Replacement Options: Failed implants may be replaced with a new implant, a bridge or a denture.

My Father's Story

My dental team members always love it when my father comes to the office for care. He is a mix of Indiana Jones, Albert Einstein, and Elmer Fudd. We know that something amusing will happen anytime he is around! Several years ago, he was eating a steak and bit a piece of bone and broke his tooth. He needed a dental implant to replace the fractured tooth. There was inadequate bone where the tooth broke, so I decided to do a sinus lift procedure to create more bone.

This was years ago -- before we had the incredible and advanced sinus techniques that we use today -- so I was using a relatively crude method of up-fracturing the bone of the sinus floor with a mallet and chisel in preparation to add bone into the sinus. Dad was peaceful and relaxed throughout the procedure.

"Clang, clang, clang" sang the hammer as I chiseled at the bone. Suddenly Dad's whole body convulsed, and he cried out in alarm! I immediately stopped and asked him what was wrong and if he was feeling any pain. "No pain," he said, "everything's fine and I don't have any pain. But I just had the craziest dream!"

He was so comfortable in the dental chair that he fell asleep while I was literally pounding on his skull with a stainless-steel hammer! Rest assured, today we have much more elegant methods and I have not used that technique for many years.

19 – DENTAL RECONSTRUCTION

My wife and I once lived in a house that was old and needed structural improvements. A quick coat of new paint and new carpets were not going to give us the results that we wanted to live with. My wife has a degree in construction management, and I love demolition, so together we tore the house apart, removed and replaced walls, retextured ceilings and replaced flooring. It was a complete remodel of the entire house. Sometimes we encounter the same thing dentally. The dental house is broken down and a few veneers or crowns are not capable of giving you the end result that you want. Sometimes we need to strip it down to the studs and remodel the entire house from scratch.

In certain situations, we can accomplish this by remodeling every tooth on one jaw. Other times it is necessary to rebuild every single tooth on both upper and lower jaws. This is required in cases with severe wear or damage due to cavities, acid erosion, clenching and grinding teeth. As with any dental treatment it is essential that the teeth have a healthy foundation of gums and bone to support the beautiful new smile. We use a combination of crowns, veneers and dental implants to build a beautiful and functional smile.

Many people that need a dental reconstruction also have issues with headaches and poor sleep. These symptoms are dramatically improved when their mouth is structurally repaired. The outcome of a dental reconstruction is a beautiful, healthy smile that supports whole body health.

Cost: Full dental reconstruction is usually charged as a comprehensive package rather than on a per-tooth basis. This can range from $20,000 to $70,000 depending on if one or both jaws are involved.

Time: Most reconstructions are done in three stages. In the diagnostic stage we put temporary crowns on the teeth to determine the proper cosmetics and fine tune the new chewing system. This usually requires 2-6 months. In the second stage we restore the front teeth with permanent crowns and veneers. In the last stage we restore the back teeth. Overall, the process can take 3-12 months to complete.

Risks: Likes other crowns and bridges, there is potential for cavities around the new dental work or fracturing the porcelain. However, in a completely remodeled smile the odds of breaking the porcelain are actually lower than in a partially restored mouth because the cause of the original broken teeth has been resolved in the new chewing system.

Maintenance: A full reconstruction is a major investment and deserves meticulous brushing and flossing at home and regular checkups at the dental office.

Life Expectancy: You can expect your new smile to need occasional updates and maintenance work after 10 to 20 years.

Replacement Options: When individual teeth have problems, they can be replaced with new crowns or bridges. If the entire reconstruction needs to be replaced the options would be another reconstruction or some form of denture.

Jose's Story

Jose was a handsome young entrepreneur, an avid hunter and a car aficionado. He came to see me because he wanted to make his smile look better. He noticed that his front teeth were chipping and wearing out unevenly. Plus, he didn't like the color of his teeth. Our routine exam revealed that Jose had a severe bite disharmony, sort of like a chair that wobbles because one leg is shorter than the others. In order to fix his broken smile, we needed to solve the problem that caused the damage in the first place -- otherwise he would break his new smile too! He asked, "Can't you just slap some veneers on my front teeth and call it good?"

I explained the likelihood of him breaking the new veneers because the problem that caused the damage to his natural teeth would still be there and I recommended that he consider a complete reconstruction to get a predictable and durable smile. I described the process of rebuilding his smile and compared it to Jose's experience of restoring one of his classic cars.

"How much is this going to cost? It sounds like as much as a new truck!" He queried.

"Yes, a very nice truck." I replied matter-of-factly.

"Dang…(long pause), Ok let's do it." he replied.

A few months later I couldn't help but smile when Jose pulled into the office for the final visit of his reconstruction driving a shiny, brand-new truck!

20 -- DENTURES

Dentures are a removable solution to replace a broken smile. Dentures can restore lost teeth as well as provide support for the lips and cheeks that has been lost due to bone shrinkage. In real estate, when you have a great piece of property but a hopelessly dilapidated building you tear down the old structure and start with a clean slate for a beautiful new building. In dentistry sometimes that's the best option as well. Often due to trauma, neglect, infection or congenital abnormalities the existing teeth cannot reasonably be modified or repaired to create a healthy, beautiful smile. In these situations, a denture is a fantastic option to replace and reconstruct the smile. Dentures have a negative stigma, but they are actually the origin of all cosmetic dentistry and a well-made denture looks every bit as beautiful as natural teeth. Thanks to modern materials, gone are the clunky wooden dentures

George Washington made famous. Patients today have a variety of options.

Partial Dentures: When some of the teeth are missing and cannot be replaced with a bridge or dental implants removable teeth (dentures) can be a great option. A removable partial denture, often called a "partial," is a little bit like a retainer that has teeth on it. It typically has a durable metal framework that supports pink gums and white teeth and uses wire clasps to hold onto the existing teeth. Partials have the advantage of being much faster and less expensive than implants. Unfortunately, partials are not as attractive as other options because the metal wires holding it in place are usually visible. If you choose to get a dental implant we can snap a partial denture on top of implant and those metal wires are longer necessary to hold the partial in place securely. A well-made partial denture should last 5-10 years and be both functional and cosmetic. You wear it during the daytime and take it out at night to clean it and allow the gums to rest.

When there are not enough teeth to help support a partial denture then we can make a full denture to replace all the teeth as well as missing bone. The bone that holds your teeth is a specialized bone, its only job is to hold your teeth. Once the teeth are gone the bone begins to melt away. Most of this bone change happens within 18 months after the teeth are removed, but it will continue slowly shrinking for the rest of your life. This loss of bone support for the lips and cheeks is noticeable in the sunken lips and cheeks of people with no teeth and without a denture. It also means that a denture may fit well initially, but over time it will need to be relined and eventually remade as the jaw shrinks. Using dental implants together with a denture can prevent bone deterioration. Implants act like natural teeth in preserving the bone so that it does not shrink or melt away.

Upper Dentures: Upper dentures typically cover the entire upper jaw, including the roof of the mouth. They are held in place largely by suction, a little bit like how a suction cup sticks to a glass window. As you chew with a full denture all of the biting forces are transferred to the gums, so while natural teeth can bite with up to 400 pounds of force, dentures typically can only bite with pressure of 40 pounds.

Upper dentures work quite well for most people as long as they have adequate bone to support the denture. Because an upper denture covers the roof of your mouth there are two unexpected changes that many patients experience when transitioning from natural teeth to a denture: speech and taste. The added thickness of the denture on the roof of your mouth will change your speech mechanics slightly. It takes time for your tongue to adapt, so it's important to be patient with yourself and allow some time for your speech to normalize. Because the denture covers the roof of the mouth it changes the way things feel when you eat. Dentures can significantly reduce the pleasure of eating as well as reducing how well you can taste your food. Both of these challenges can be avoided through the use of dental implants as described below.

Lower Dentures: While upper dentures work pretty well for most people, lower dentures are another story. Instead of having a broad footprint to cover the entire jaw, lower dentures are a horseshoe shape that sits on top of a narrow jawbone and wraps around the tongue. This eliminates the potential for suction to hold the denture in place (have you ever seen a horseshoe shaped suction cup? Me either!) and lower dentures are much less stable than upper dentures. While they work well for many of my patients, I always warn patients to be prepared for some frustration and challenges with the lower denture because they are nowhere near as satisfying as upper dentures. However, this situation can be resolved by adding dental implants.

Transitioning to a Denture: There are two routes to get to a beautiful new smile with dentures: toothless and immediate.

For ideal cosmetics and fit we fabricate the denture while there are no teeth in the jaw so that we can do multiple try-on visits and fine-tuning -- customizing the denture exactly to your preferences. This usually takes four to six visits over about four weeks. However, it also means that if you don't already have a denture to wear in the meantime, you'll be toothless for about a month!

If you have existing teeth that need to be removed, then we create a denture called an immediate denture. With this method we make copies of your teeth beforehand and fabricate the denture based off the position of your existing teeth, accounting for any cosmetic improvements you want. At the second visit we remove your existing teeth and put in your new denture teeth all in the same visit. With this method you never have to go without teeth. The disadvantage is that we cannot try the denture on beforehand so we cannot fine-tune the cosmetics or the fit. I usually recommend that patients use an immediate denture as a steppingstone toward a second denture. One or two years after the extractions the bone will have stabilized and you can get a new denture with ideal fit and cosmetics, while keeping your first denture as a backup in case of an emergency.

Removable Implant Dentures: For almost every patient we can place implants into the upper or lower jaw and then the denture can snap onto the implants. This works similar to snaps on a shirt or a trailer hitch ball on a pickup truck. With the implants in place the denture becomes dramatically more stable. With an upper denture snapped onto implants we no longer need the roof of the mouth to provide suction, so we can create a horseshoe-shaped upper denture that keeps your abilities of speech and taste while the implants keep the denture securely in place. When using dental implants to secure a removable denture we need at least two implants on the lower jaw and four implants on the upper jaw.

Removable implant dentures are easy to clean. Every day you should snap out the denture to clean it and brush and clean your implants. Dental implants have radically changed patients' perspectives on dentures and provide a tremendous amount of security and peace of mind. *You no longer need to worry about your denture flying out of your mouth when you cough, sing, or go skydiving!*

Permanent Implant Dentures: If you need the cosmetics and function of a denture with the security and confidence of natural teeth a permanent denture is the best option. A permanent denture is a full set of teeth that is permanently connected to four or more dental implants. It can only be removed in the dental office -- at home you brush and clean your teeth in your mouth just like you would with natural teeth. This option has become very popular in recent years and it is sometimes called "teeth in a day," "All-on-4," or a "hybrid denture." Like an immediate denture, this method allows us to make sure that you never go without teeth. You come in with your natural teeth, we remove the teeth, we place the implants, and we connect the permanent denture all in the same visit. This actually requires more than just one day because there are multiple office visits to plan and make the denture in advance; so, don't expect to come in for a consultation and walk out with a full set of new teeth on implants that same afternoon!

After the initial surgery and placement of the preliminary denture we let the implants heal for six months. After the implants have successfully healed, we remove the preliminary denture and place the final denture. We can make cosmetic changes at that time. Permanent dentures have radically improved the lives and smiles of many patients, they are a remarkable advancement in dentistry.

Cost: Partial dentures and removable full dentures typically start at $2,000. Implant snap-on dentures cost between $10,000 and $20,000. Permanent dentures cost up to $30,000 per jaw.

Time: Removable dentures and partials take four to six weeks to fabricate. Immediate dentures can be ready within one week. Permanent dentures can be ready within three to six weeks with a second phase of treatment six months later.

Risks: A partial denture relies on the adjacent teeth for support and it can apply extra forces to those teeth, so if the gums are infected or the teeth are weak the partial can cause damage to (or loss of) neighboring teeth. The primary risk for a removable denture is the instability and insecurity of losing suction and having the denture fall out at an inconvenient moment.

Dentures that rely on implants risk the implant failing or becoming infected. All types of dentures have the potential to fracture or break.

The #1 cause of broken dentures for my patients is dogs chewing on them, so keep them safe from little Fido!

Maintenance: Partials and removable dentures must be taken out and cleaned every single day and the underlying teeth, gums, or implants must also be maintained daily at home, as well as routine hygiene visits at the dental office. Permanent dentures are brushed and flossed in your mouth just like natural teeth and need professional cleaning at the dental office twice a year. If you want to avoid additional maintenance as much as possible a basic removable denture is the best option.

Life Expectancy: Removable dentures can be expected to last 5 to 10 years, Permanent dentures should last 10-20 years before repair or replacement is needed.

Replacement Options: Any denture can be replaced with a new denture.

Gertrude's Story

Gertrude and Bernard were a delightful couple in their 80's that I have been treating for many years. They had been married for almost 60 years and Bernard treated Gertrude like a queen. Every time she came to the office, he would walk her back to the treatment room, get her settled, and then go wait out in the reception area while she got her dental work done. What he did not know was that she had worn a denture since before they got married!

Bubba's Story

The first patient I ever made a denture for was a tall, skinny man who called himself Bubba. He had ugly, gnarled teeth and he wanted a smile that was "so bright that when I smile you have to put on shades!" I made him a beautiful, bright white denture that he loved. But when he came back for his follow-up visit, he was disappointed.

"I can't eat as fast with my dentures as I could before" he whined. "My wife can eat three Big Macs in the time that I can eat one. Without my dentures I could eat a Big Mac in two bites!"

I told Bubba that I thought it was probably a good thing for him to slow down and eat with his dentures in!

21 – NON-TRADITIONAL COSMETICS

Although most people want straight, pearly white teeth, there are the number of other treatments that some people find cosmetic. I've had requests for things that I do not find cosmetic, but patients are absolutely thrilled by, including: crowns with special designs like four leaf clovers, Mercedes-Benz symbols, peace signs, and black and white spots like a cow. Beauty is in the eye of the beholder and I am happy to help with whatever makes you happy, as long as it is not harmful to your health. The only service that I've refused to do for a patient was to do root canals on all of his perfectly healthy teeth then file them down to pointed fangs.

Beauty is in the eye of the beholder!

Brandon's Story

Brandon came to my office with one specific request: "I want gold on my two front teeth." His teeth were healthy, straight and white and looked great to me, but he wanted some bling. Together we planned to place gold veneers on his two front teeth and he began coming in every week and making cash payments in preparation for his treatment.

When he had finally saved up enough to pay for the two front teeth, he changed his mind and decided that he wanted to do four teeth instead of just two. Several more weeks passed as he diligently came in and made his payments every Friday.

Soon he was finally ready to begin. We made the gold veneers and I placed them on his teeth, concerned about how he would feel seeing so much gold in his formerly white smile. I handed him the mirror, upon which he said Oh #%&*... (long pause) ... I should have done all six teeth!"

Diamond Teeth

Sandra was a middle-aged woman with a healthy, beautiful smile but she wanted something a little more exciting in her life. She asked if I could put a diamond on her tooth. At the time I thought that was a terrible idea and tried to talk her out of it, but she was absolutely insistent on getting a diamond on her tooth. I made her sign a disclaimer absolving me of all responsibility for how it looked and then I bonded a real diamond on her upper right cuspid. To my astonishment it looked fantastic! Within days two of my employees also got diamonds on their teeth.

Several years later my partner and I put fake diamonds on each other's teeth before a team meeting as a joke. The team found our glittering smiles terribly distracting and teased us relentlessly.

When I got home my wife immediately noticed my glinting tooth and said, "You look silly, go take that thing off."

When my partner got home his wife said, "That's amazing, when do I get mine?"

Part 3

Bonus Material

Shane Sykes, DMD

22 – HOW TO CHOOSE A DENTIST

Little known questions every patient should ask before choosing a dentist.

Some relationships require a lot more trust than others. Do you have a weak relationship with your grocery store clerk? No big deal. A bad relationship with your hairdresser? Absolutely a big deal! Trust and connection become more important when we're seeking service from someone who comes inside our "personal space" and for Americans, that bubble is about three feet. When someone comes inside our personal space they're generally either coming in for a kiss or to land a punch. Most patients don't feel like I'm going to kiss them! So finding a dentist with whom you have a strong relationship of trust is very important.

The first place to look for a dentist is a referral from trusted friends who already have a dentist they love. They've already done the detective work and can tell you about their relationship with their dentist. In today's socially connected world the next best thing to a referral from a friend is public reviews. Read the reviews for any dental office you are interested in. Beyond just the star-rating of the reviews, what is the content of those reviews? Are there sincere reviews from patients? Some bad reviews are to be expected, so an office that only has 5-star ratings may be a little suspicious. Use the experience of others to help you get a head start on the relationship with your new dentist.

Making the Call:

Once you narrow it down to a few offices to call, here are some key questions you can ask over the phone before you make a dental appointment. These five questions will help you find the right dentist for you:

1. What continuing education has the dentist taken in the last 12 months? New developments in dentistry are emerging every day. Leading edge technologies, new ways to diagnose, and better treatments are being discovered, tested, and confirmed regularly. You want a dentist who is keeping up with all of the newest developments and who knows all of the potential treatments for every condition. State requirements, however, are minimal to maintain a license to practice dentistry. For instance, in Indiana a dentist is only required to have 10 hours of continuing education each year. That's less than a single workday for some people! Is the dentist just doing the minimum required to stay in practice are they or striving to stay educated so you will stay healthy? If the appointment coordinator on the phone can't tell you what seminars the dentist has taken lately, it is likely that there haven't been very many!

2. How long will it take to perform my initial examination? Be sure that you are going to a dentist who will provide a thorough exam so that you and the dentist will be totally aware of your entire oral health condition. Check to see if the dentist will take the time with you to discuss your condition and treatment options. If you want comprehensive care, you don't want to go to an office where the dentist comes in for 15 seconds then runs off to see another patient. A thorough dentist will set aside at least an hour or more to do a complete exam and consultation.

3. What is included in my initial exam? Some dentists just take a cursory glance around and ask what hurts. This may be a "look-see" to detect the obvious, but it isn't an effective exam that will protect you and your long-term health. You want a relationship in which the dentist and their team take the time to get to know you personally and learn what is important to you so they can make appropriate recommendations for your health. There are four things a thorough exam should include:

(a) A check of all your teeth for decay including the current condition of any existing restorations. Notes should be made on your chart of all existing restorations and the condition of all of your other teeth. You should be given the option of having a full series of X-Rays rather that whatever limited x-rays your insurance will cover if the total condition of your dental health is being evaluated thoroughly.

(b) A complete and thorough check of the health of your gums with a periodontal probe. This is a tiny ruler used to measure the gums and bone around each tooth. Six points on every tooth should be checked and the findings charted every single year.

(c) A check of your bite should be made to determine how your teeth come together. The check should determine if there is balance, excessive wear, or jaw pain.

(d) There should be a detailed exam and discussion to check for any signs of oral cancer, sleep apnea, dietary concerns or other whole-body health issues that have signs or symptoms that show up in the mouth. Because most people see their dentist far more often than their physician, you want a dentist who takes the time to help keep your whole body healthy.

4. Ask what will occur between the time of your arrival at the office and when the dentist starts the actual exam. This will determine if there will be time for you to talk to a treatment coordinator or to the dentist before the work begins. A dentist interested in you and your health will set time aside to listen to your concerns and expectations during your first visit.

5. Ask when the dental team went through Occupational Safety and Health Administration (OSHA) compliance training. OSHA has very clear guidelines for dental offices to follow in order to maintain the highest standard of sterilization and infection control. Every member of the dental office team is required by law to take compliance training at least once a year.

When you have investigated these five things, take time to do a brief mental review of the experience you have had. Recall how you have been treated on the phone. Because the attitudes in the office trickle down from the top, the treatment you receive from the appointment coordinator can often be an indication of how you are going to be treated in that office by other team members and the dentist.

Your First Visit:

After you've selected a dentist to visit, your research is not done. As you enter the office, be a detective. You may see little things that could be symptoms of more significant things going on behind the scenes. Here are some things to observe:

1. Is the reception area tidy, organized, neat, and clean? How about the patient restroom nearest the reception area? What you find there will likely give you an idea of what you can expect in the total office in terms of organization, cleanliness, and attention to detail.

2. Are you seen on time? This will provide an indication of whether this is a people-oriented practice or one that is just treating teeth. It may not be realistic to expect the dental practice to be right on schedule all the time, but it is realistic to expect to be told within 10 minutes of your arrival if there will be a time delay.

3. Are the doctor and the members of the dental team good examples of proper dental health and hygiene? Do they have attractive smiles? This is an indication of whether they believe in what they are doing. The dental team members should be good examples of the service they provide. If the optimal dental health you want for yourself is not important enough to the providers you have chosen to have it done for themselves, then there is reason to question the recommendations you might be given by those providers.

4. How is the relationship among the dental team members? Is it a respectful, harmonious environment where people enjoy what they do and whom they work with? Or will your providers be distracted by a toxic environment and not be able to give you their best?

The above suggestions are just some of the things you can ask and observe in order to make the right choice of a dentist who will serve you and your needs the best. Take the time to ask the right questions so you'll have the peace of mind of knowing that you are in the best hands for what you want for the long-term health of your mouth and your smile.

Vanessa's Husband's Story

Vanessa has been a patient in my office for several years and we had a great relationship. Unfortunately, her husband Mike was deathly afraid of the dentist (I know, I'm a pretty intimidating guy!) and he had never been into our office. Once day he had a terrible toothache that had been keeping him awake for four days but he refused to go to the dentist. Vanessa called and asked if I could help, of course I said I would be happy to see Mike.

We scheduled an emergency visit for Mike to see me, but when they arrived for his appointment she leaned over the check-in counter and whispered to the receptionist that she lied to him and told him she needed to pick something up at our office and asked if he would come along with her. Talk about a bait and switch! I was stuck in the awkward position of trying to transition from a pretend visit for Vanessa to providing care for the unsuspecting yet supportive husband that just got duped into stepping into a dental office for the first time in 25 years.

Fortunately we were able to sit down with the three of us together and visit about her dental health, their children and her pregnancy, and eventually I was able to ask about his dental health and he admitted that he did have a toothache. We were not able to provide treatment to solve his pain at that visit, but we were able to break down the barrier of fear and anxiety that prevented him from coming in. A few days later he walked into the office timidly but of his own volition and we were able to make him comfortable and solve his pain.

23 – MAXIMIZING YOUR DENTAL INSURANCE

Many patients are fortunate to have dental insurance to help pay for their needs. This can be a tremendous help in maintaining your health, Unfortunately, dental insurance is not designed to help you *become* healthy, but rather to help you *stay* healthy. In 1978, the year I was born, the average dental insurance provided $1,000 of dental coverage and a dental crown cost $200. Today the average dental insurance still provides $1,000 of dental coverage but the average crown costs $1,500. That's a 4% annual increase in dental fees *without any insurance increase at all over more than four decades!*

Perplexingly, dental insurance is not actually *insurance*, it is a *rebate*. With most medical insurances the patient pays the first few thousand dollars and the medical insurance takes care of everything after that. Dental insurance is the opposite. Dental insurance might reimburse a portion of the first $1,000, and the patient pays everything else after that. So it's important to not let your dental insurance dictate your healthcare, but instead use it as a tool to help accelerate and improve your oral health without getting in the way of the care that you want and need. One of the best ways to maximize your benefits is to make sure that you're actually using all of your benefits. Get your regular checkups and cleanings at least twice a year, and if you have treatment needs, they can sometimes be planned to be spread over two years to take advantage of both years benefits.

David's Story

My patient David is a very busy investment banker, father and little-league coach. Shortly before Christmas David's tooth started hurting and suddenly, he realized he hadn't been to our dental office in *five years*! As an investment guru she was suddenly painfully aware that meant he had not used his dental benefits for five years even though he had been paying for them! He was furious with himself for wasting that money and called our office pained not only by his tooth but also by the dental insurance money he had wasted. He was desperate for help and we were booked solid through the end of the year, but we made special arrangements and invited him into the office right away. We were able to help him take advantage of the benefits he had remaining for that year as well as make a plan to get his smile healthy and make sure he didn't waste any benefits in the years to come. Now he makes sure that he always schedules his next appointment before he leaves the office, and he has not wasted a dime of his dental benefits since!

24 – SEEKING DENTISTRY ABROAD

There's no doubt about it, sophisticated dentistry is a significant investment. Because of the cost of dentistry, many people are interested in seeking dental care overseas where they can get work done at a much lower cost than in the United States. And who can blame them? If you can get the exact same care in India for one-tenth the US price, why not? If you wanted a full set of upper and lower Teeth in a Day in the US that would cost about $60,000, but you can get the same procedure in Thailand for $16,000, and you can make a fantastic vacation out of it! Of course, that all depends on if you can get the same quality of care.

I have treated a number of patients that have received dental care overseas and I have seen wonderful outcomes. Unfortunately, I have also seen tragic complications. I am not at all opposed to patients seeking care abroad, just make sure are well informed and know what you're getting into.

for one tenth of one ounce, or $16,000 per pound. However, you can go to Home Depot and grab a hefty 47-pound bag of Portland Cement (almost chemically identical to MTA) for a mere twenty-six cents per pound! Dental products in the US cost a lot. Overseas they can buy things much cheaper, but they are not held to the same standards of fabrication as products intended for the United States market. Additionally, even though they may use the same manufacturers they are not getting exactly the same products, or if they are they're called by different names. For example, I had a patient that went to Costa Rica to have an implant placed and then came to me to put the crown on top of the implant. The Costa Rica dentist used an implant brand that I also use, but the particular model of implant he used is not available in the US and we had to order the abutment and crown parts from overseas. Ultimately, we got it done but it took a few months longer than needed and required a lot of back and forth for the patient to track down the parts.

Before you fully commit to treatment overseas make sure you understand exactly what will be required, how many visits and how long you'll need to be there each time. Do lots of research and make sure you are comfortable with the provider you are visiting. Try to find unfiltered patient reviews, and don't rely solely on before/after photos or testimonials that have been carefully curated by the dentist. This applies to dental care locally as well!

Emily's Story

Emily loved had yoga and decided to move to India for a year to pursue training to be a yogi. She had some pretty bad dental problems and could not afford the dentistry that she wanted in the USA. While she was in India she decided to have all of her teeth removed and 16 dental implants placed. Porcelain bridges were used to replace all of her teeth. Three years later she came to me for help because her teeth felt a little bit loose. When I looked in her mouth I was horrified. Although I recognized the implant hardware used and knew it to be a quality product, the dentist had violated nearly all the rules of implant success. I had to give her the bad news that for me to fix her implants would cost over $35,000. In her efforts to save money she actually ended up spending far more.

Amanda's Story

Amanda previously had all her teeth removed and beautiful dentures made by her local dentist. Unfortunately, she had a terrible gag reflex and her dentures made her so nauseous she could only stand to wear them for brief stints for family pictures. She was a young mother and the lack of teeth was destroying her self-esteem. We discussed the options of dental implants to support permanent dentures. We went through an extensive treatment planning process diagnosing exactly what her options were and how we would move forward with it. I was surprised when she contacted me two weeks later asking if I could take her stitches out. "We haven't done anything yet, why do you have stitches?" I asked. She explained that she went to Mexico and had the exact same procedure done there instead and wondered if I could do all of her follow-up visits. When I saw her to remove the sutures, I was concerned by what I saw and prescribed antibiotics and mouth rinses to treat the infection present. It remains yet to be seen whether or not she will be able to salvage her implants.

REFERENCES

1 - Harker, L. & Keltner, D., (2001). Expressions of Positive Emotion in WOmen's College Yearbook Pictures and THeir Relationship to Personality and Life Outcomes Across Adulthood. *Journal of Personality and Social Psychology*, Vol. 80, No. 1, 112-124

2 - Abel, E. L., Kruger, M. L., (2010). Smile Intensity in Photographs Predicts Longevity. *Psychological Science,* 21 (4) 542-544.

3 - Valente, D., et. al. (2018). The Role of Visual Experience in the Production of Emotional Facial Expressions by Blind People: A Review, *Psychonomic Bulletin & Review*, 25 (2) 483-497.

4 - Ekman, P. (1971). Universals and Cultural Differences in Facial Expressions of Emotion. *Nebraska Symposium on Motivation,* 19 207-282.

5 - Provine, R. R., (2001). *Laughter: A Scientific Investigation.* Penguin paperback.

6 - Dimberg, U., Thunberg, M., Elmehed, K., (2000). Unconscious Facial Reactions to Emotional Facial Expressions. *Psychological Science,* 11 (1) 86-89.

7 - Rychlowska, M., et. al. (2014). Blocking Mimicry Makes True and False Smiles Look the Same, *Plos One*, 9 (3)

8 - Hennenlotter, A., et. al. (2019) The Link Between Facial Feedback and Neural Activity within Central Circuitries of Emotion - New Insights from Botulinum Toxin-induced Denervation of Frown Muscles. *Cerebral Cortex,* 19 (3) 237-542.

References

9 - Kraft, T. L., Pressman, S. D. (2012) Grin and Bear It: The Influence of Manipulated Facial Expression on the Stress Response. *Psychological Sciences,* 23 (11) 1372-1378.

10 - Refer to Susan Harter's comprehensive work on Self-Perception (University of Denver).

11 - Grandey, A. A., et. al. (2019). When Are Fakers Also Drinkers? A Self-Control View of Emotional Labor and Alcohol Consumption Among U.S. Service Workers. *Journal of Occupational Health Psychology,* 24 (4) 482-497.

12 - Grammer, K., Thornhill, R. (1994). Human (Homo Sapiens) Facial Attractiveness and Sexual Selection: The Role of Symmetry and Averageness. *Journal of Comparative Psychology,* 108 (3) 233-242

13 - Machado, A. W., (2014). 10 Commandments of Smile Esthetics. *Dental Press Journal of Orthodontics,* 19 (4) 136-157.

14 - LaMonte, M. J., et. al. (2017). History of Periodontitis Diagnosis and Edentulism as Predictors of Coardiovascular Diseae, Stroke, and Mortality in Postmenopausal Women. *Journal of the American Heart Association,* 6 (4).

ABOUT THE AUTHOR

Dr. Shane Sykes practices General Dentistry in Reno, Nevada. While studying at Brigham Young University and the University of Kentucky he excelled in both clinical and psychological sciences, receiving numerous scholarships and awards. Dr. Sykes has practiced dentistry in Idaho, Utah, Alaska, and Nevada. Some devoted patients travel across the country to continue receiving their dental care from Dr. Sykes. He enjoys providing humanitarian dental service both locally and overseas.

Because Dr. Sykes has lived and worked in some of the world's poorest and wealthiest communities, he has developed understanding and love for people in all walks of life. His dental artistry stems from his lifelong love of art

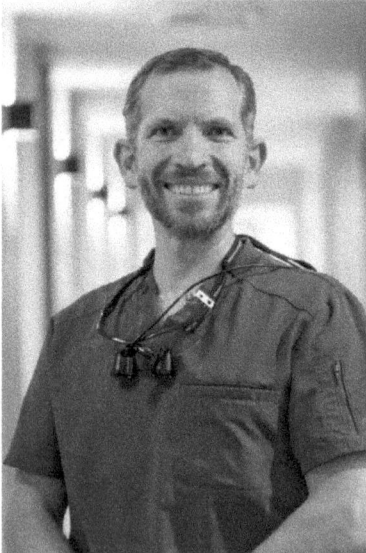

and photography, while his practical approach to dental care comes through his experiences in psychology, teaching and problem solving.

Shane, his wife, and their six young children enjoy a rural lifestyle. As a family they have lived on bicycles for nine months, climbed Africa's highest peak, raised Tibetan yaks, and trained wild mustangs.